T0199026

Vege Kick

MEENA MISTRY

Balboa Press books may be ordered through booksellers or by contacting:

Balboa Press
A Division of Hay House
1663 Liberty Drive
Bloomington, IN 47403
www.balboapress.com
844-682-1282

ISBN: 978-1-9822-5161-1 (sc)
ISBN: 978-1-9822-5162-8 (e)

Library of Congress Control Number: 2020913574

Print information available on the last page.

Balboa Press rev. date: 08/17/2020

BALBOA.PRESS
A DIVISION OF HAY HOUSE

DEDICATIONS

This book is a special dedication to my daughters Kunjal and Neera. Their enthusiasm, inspiration, unreserved love and support has given me an unwavering encouragement and motivation to take on this new challenge and excitement to fulfill my dreams with a view to sharing some of the best ideas and recipes based on vegetarian ingredients for people to enjoy.

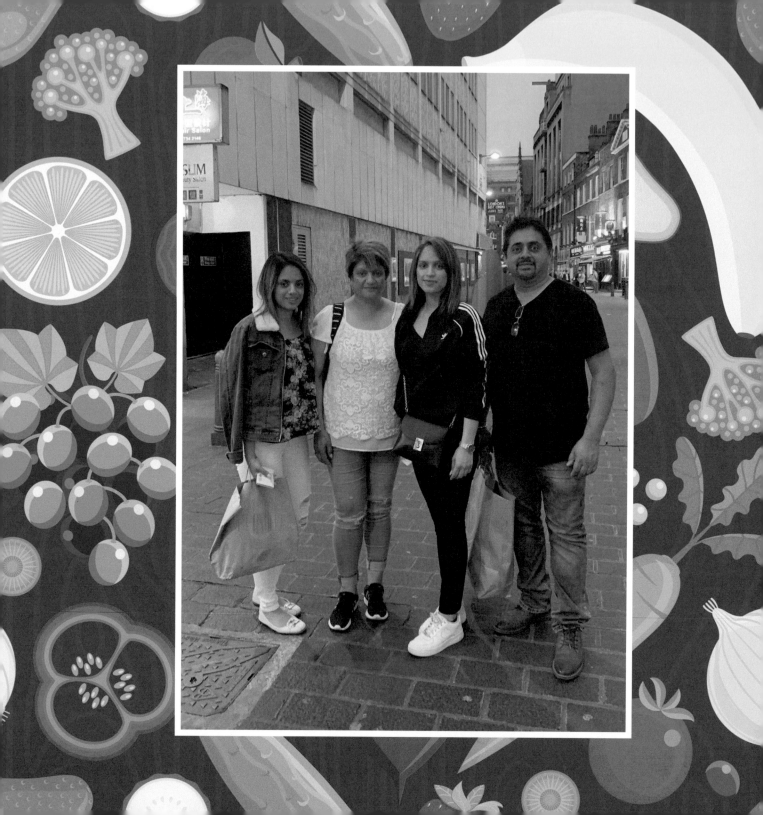

ACKNOWLEDGEMENTS

Cooking and creating recipes have been my passion for many years. My interest in the culinary world took a much more positive turn during my stay in England, U.K. for many years. The joy of cooking evolved dramatically through the effective use of herbs and spices for diversified vegetarian cooking. This led to a unique exposure and experience within a school system catering program and its associated students' healthy eating practice of having a balanced meal inclusive of a variety of vegetables.

I strongly believe that eating vegetables as a complementary option to non-vegetarian foods is an optimized and wholistic solution for a healthy diet. In 2006 I moved to the United States where I continued to conjure up and develop unique ideas for tasty vegetation dishes for my family and friends to enjoy. I had to come up with recipes which took relatively shorter time to put the food on the table and potentially interesting to eat. This eventually led me to writing my first book "Spicy N Easy" which was published in 2012. This text reflected my enthusiasm, passion and love of culinary skills of vegetarian cooking through unique section of spices, herbs and vegetables.

Living in the State of Illinois brought a pleasant surprise for me in the world of food. I was approached by a local high school district with a view to talking about healthy eating through demonstrating recipes in the school kitchen. This initiative was being exercised through the school teachers wellbeing program. Getting involved in this initiative was very exciting but more importantly confirmed my belief and passion that vegetarian foods have a unique and important place in the culinary world from health and taste perspectives.

My close friend Jennifer Johnson, her husband Randy and daughter Rebecca and many others have given me a lot of support and many positive feedbacks on the taste of the food that I have made over the last few years. More importantly this has given me a further sense of purpose and drive to continually develop more recipes and unique ways of cooking for my family and friends to enjoy.

Vege Kick offers a different and unique approach for combining spices, herbs and vegetarian ingredients for creating dishes in a way that will leave a person with great satisfaction upon eating the prepared meal. I strongly believe that this text will find its place in many households. Please enjoy!

Lastly, I would like to thank my husband Anuj for his continued support. Thank you.

Meena Mistry

VEGE KICK: TABLE OF CONTENTS

INTRODUCTION

Vegetarian cooking is an art that requires skill and perfection. Asian and Indian vegetarian food has evolved over thousands of years, although through geographical migration and transformation cooking skills have diversified to cater for different background people globally.

Individuals choosing to follow a vegetarian diet often choose additional healthy lifestyle habits such as regular physical exercise, frequent exposure to sunlight and fresh air. These are all factors considered essential to achieving and maintaining balanced health and a healthy body weight.

A healthy vegetarian diet is one in which a variety and abundance of plant-based foods such as grains, legumes, vegetables, herbs and spices are primarily eaten. Most meals comprise of several dishes ranging from appetizers, rice, lentils, breads, and vegetables. I must not forget to mention that vegetables are usually complemented with a selection of breads. These include "nan" bread and its various derivatives.

We often ask ourselves and others what makes individuals to follow vegetarianism. There are many reasons for this. One common one is through inheritance within an extended family which was quite often the case generations ago in families. In modern times, vegetarianism has become a way of living through reasons of health, self-awareness, cultural awareness, taste and ethnicity.

There are many definitions of vegetarianism that exist in the culinary world, however, the definition of vegetarianism that has formed the basis of this book is based on plant-based ingredients that resulted into selected recipes and meals.

Cooking has taken a delicate and intricate art of blending herbs and spices with base stocks for perfection in the culinary world. In my opinion food can include perhaps the most dazzling array of fresh vegetables cooked in a multitude of ways that help retain their freshness, nutrients and more importantly the resulting taste on that serving plate.

All lentils and pulses are nutritious and play an important part in vegetarian diet. They are excellent sources of fibre and protein and are low in cholesterol and fat. Additionally, lentils and pulses are extremely easy to prepare. Consider the use of moong beans. Sprouted or not, moong beans form excellent curries and other quick meals such as salads.

Soya has played a role in many foods. Soya products that originate from the bean "soya bean". This has been the source of protein in Asia for many years and is no secret that it has been a significant part of vegetarian diet. Soya has additionally presented itself as a good alternative to dairy product and has also been accepted as a useful alternative to meat for vegetarians. I have demonstrated the use of soya through various creative preparations that the readers of this book will find interesting and tasty.

The use of herbs and spices like turmeric, ginger, garlic, green chillies and many more has continued to evolve over the years for their flavour and aroma. It is fun and beneficial that that one understands what these typical herbs and spices are and what effects they have.

A BRIEF LOOK AT HERBS AND SPICES

Herbs and spices form an important part of vegetarian cooking and is a must in every kitchen. How does an herb differ from a spice? Herbs are essentially plant fresh leaves or fall in the category of powdered dried leaves. It is a plant whose stem does not produce and woody persistent tissue and generally dies back at the end of each growing season.

Spices result from seeds, roots, berries and certain stems and usually native to warm tropical climates. These are dried and used in powder or ground form or whole. It is the volatile oils in the herbs and spices that provide some of the useful properties namely flavoring, aroma, preservation and medicinal that are beneficial in culinary.

Trying to understand herbs and species and the importance of their correct use will take the person in the kitchen a long way in perfecting the art of vegetarian cooking.

The key to using herbs and spices is to optimize the flavouring in the foods that will be prepared for the consumer and it is no secret and is common sense to use freshly prepared herbs and spices in the kitchen. The question still remains in our minds as to how much to use.

The secret of a successful and a tasty recipe is significantly contributed by such ingredients. While they give a flavour and aroma to the food being cooked it is the right combination of them which makes the overall contribution to the recipe. Herbs and spices not only give that desired taste to the food, they are also reported to provide positive medicinal effects on the body.

Vegetarian cooking is an art and a skill that can be mastered and perfected by anyone who dedicates to this learning. The secret ingredient to a tasty vegetarian dish is the knowledge of spices, the herbs and their right combination nurtured by the very person in the kitchen.

The secret of success in using the spices and herbs lies in the way they are combined and blended. It is fun working with items such as bay leaves, nutmeg, black pepper, coriander, cinnamon, cardamom and cloves when preparing food and targeting those taste buds.

Herbs and spices have a potent effect on the food and are used sparingly and as needed for developing the unique and optimized flavors of the dishes. It will be interesting to review key spices and herbs of which some have been used in the recipes.

Coriander is used as an add-on spice to enhance flavoring and is commonly found both as whole dried seeds and in powder form. Seeds may be heated on a dry pan briefly before grinding to enhance and alter the aroma. The seeds are shaped as tiny balls and they give that distinctive spicy sweet flavor. They are used as a flavoring for food and as a seasoning as well as in curries and curry powder.

Cilantro is essentially coriander leaves which have a sage-citrus flavor and an almost pungent aroma. Chopped cilantro is used for seasoning and garnishing and is very popular in Latin American and Asian foods. It is always best to use fresh cilantro when using for culinary seasoning since its aroma is optimized.

Cumin is a dried seed of the parsley family. Cumin is used as a spice for its distinctive peppery aroma and is very popular in India and Asian cuisines. This is an essential ingredient for preparing vegetarian curries and many appetizers in whole or ground form.

Chilies are used fresh green or red and in powder form for most preparations to provide a unique flavor and hotness in the food. Quite often one wants to have the chili flavor but without that hotness. In this case one can remove the seeds from the whole chili and add the rest becomes part of the ingredients in finely chopped form. It is wise to use chilies sparingly during cooking. Sometimes may decide to put chili powder in ready cooked food to give additional hotness.

Cinnamon is primarily used as a condiment and provides a distinct pungent sweet flavoring. Cinnamon grows as brown bark which upon drying, rolls into a tubular form. Cinnamon can be bought either its whole form (sticks) or as ground powder. Cinnamon sticks are quite often used in preparing rice dishes and various dal soups.

Cloves are dried buds of the clove tree. Cloves are used as a spice in cuisines all over the world to give that unique almost bitter sweet flavor. They can be used in cooking either whole or in a ground form. Use cloves in small amounts since they are extremely are used sparingly.

Garlic has a characteristic pungent, spicy flavor that mellows extremely well with cooking as a condiment. Its intense aroma and health benefits certainly make a mark in the food it is used in.

Ginger is a rhizome tuber that is frequently used to provide a peppery sweet flavor and preservative capabilities. For best results and effectiveness it is very wise to use freshly grated ginger when preparing foods. It provides excellent aroma and taste when used for a number of dishes such lentils, pulses and tikka varieties.

Mustard seeds have a special place in culinary and is often used for garnishing during which the seeds are quickly and lightly fried in oil as a prerequisite for curry and similar and similar dish preparations. Mustard seeds provide a pungent, nutty but a nutritious flavoring.

Turmeric is part of the ginger family that has found itself uniquely in Asian and Persian cuisines for its taste, reported medicinal and coloring ability. It gives a warm and aromatic flavors when used in correct amount.

The health benefits of herbs and spices are widely known and reported. I have been very fortunate to be in a position to witness and experience most of these benefits and to be able to associate these with creation of my recipes. Spices can be useful and be beneficial if used correctly and in right proportions.

Cilantro and cumin are known to assist in digestion, flatulence and upset stomach. They are also sources of iron and magnesium.

Cumin aids in digestion, common cold, anemia, skin disorders additionally boost our immune system.

Chilies, in moderation, contribute significantly when it comes to aiding health. They are known to prevent sinusitis and help remove mucus from your nose and relieve congestion. Additionally, chilies help combat inflammation and soothe intestinal diseases. Chilies are potentially thermogenic and they assist in fat metabolism resulting in increased body heat.

Cinnamon equally is beneficial to our dietary habits. Various benefits of cinnamon have been reported. These include lowering of cholesterol, regulate blood sugar, anti-clotting effecting on blood and acts like a natural food preservative and is a good source of fiber, manganese, calcium and iron.

Clove and clove oil have successfully been used for toothaches, respiratory problems, and indigestion and as an antiseptic. Clove oil is also known to assist with blood circulation and purification. Cloves contain manganese, omega 3 fatty acids, vitamins K and C and fiber and are a good all-round health supplement.

The potential benefits of Garlic are reportedly more pronounced and effective when eaten freshly chopped or crushed and in moderation. Garlic has been known to help with cardiovascular and high cholesterol conditions.

Ginger appears to help fight morning sickness, reduce pain and inflammation. It is also reported to help relieve heart burn, motion sickness, cold and flu.

Mustard is one of the most popular spices and contributes significantly as a beneficial source of nutritional health. It contains omega-3 fatty acids, iron, fiber and other minerals. It has the ability to be stimulating digestion.

Turmeric is probably one of the most powerful spices which has found its use in many cultures. The inherent health benefits of turmeric have gradually surfaced over hundreds of years. It has successfully been used in Asia for its anti-inflammatory properties, wound healing, skin disorders and many more.

The idea to review the benefits is to bring an awareness and realization of how these benefits can be successfully incorporated in cooking, especially in vegetarian cooking.

Being vegetarian has its potential proven benefits but to compliment vegetables and ingredients classed as vegetarian with spices and herbs that were discussed earlier, takes a relatively new prospective as part of healthy life style.

Rice finds itself uniquely embedded in many cultures as well. Rice of different grain type is grown as a staple crop across the globe especially in East and South Asia, the Middle East, South America, and West Indies. While having a nutritional value for a balanced meal, rice can be cooked in a number of ways.

In this day and age vegetables, herbs, species and vegetarian based products are found in abundance and in almost every corner of the world. Vegetarianism has become a way of life for many people for multiple reasons.

My personal approach to cooking through a unique selection of herbs, spices and vegetarian based ingredients and turning them into quick and enjoyable recipes, which some of them are vegan, will be of great interest and value to readers of this book, their friends, their family members and colleagues.

For fun and taste I have also included a couple of desserts so let us indulge in some of the recipes in my kitchen and turn them to yours to enjoy.......

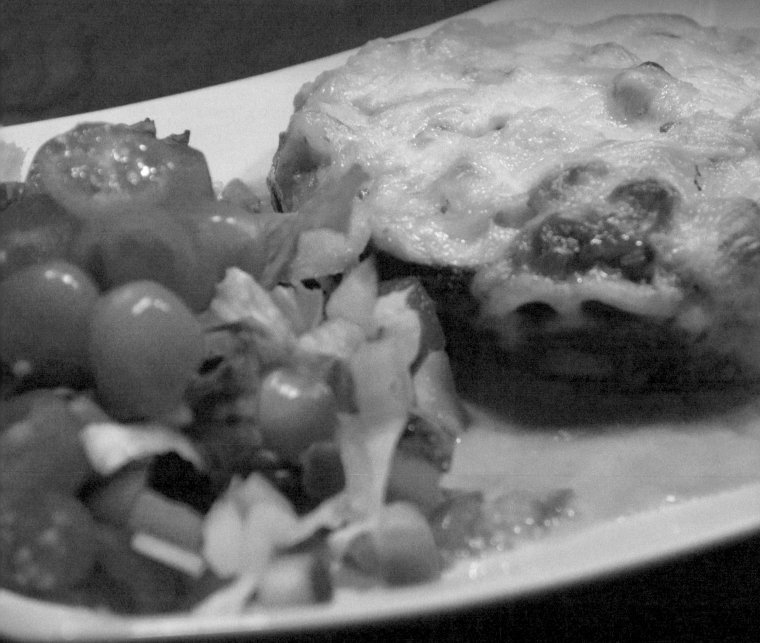

Stuffed Portobello

Ingredients

2 large portobello mushrooms
1 cup chopped small mushrooms
white sauce (refer to recipe in this book)
1 cup grated cheddar cheese

Procedure

1. Place two mushrooms in an ovenproof tray, top them with chopped mushrooms, white sauce and grated cheddar cheese.
2. Bake at 400 °F for 15-20 minutes or until golden brown.

Serves 2

White Sauce

Ingredients

2½ cups milk
¼ cup butter
1 tsp English mustard
¼ cup all-purpose white flour
1 cup water
½ cup cheese

Procedure

1. In a pan, add milk, butter, mustard and bring to boil.
2. In a separate container add water, flour, mix well and slowly add to the pan making sure there are no lumps.

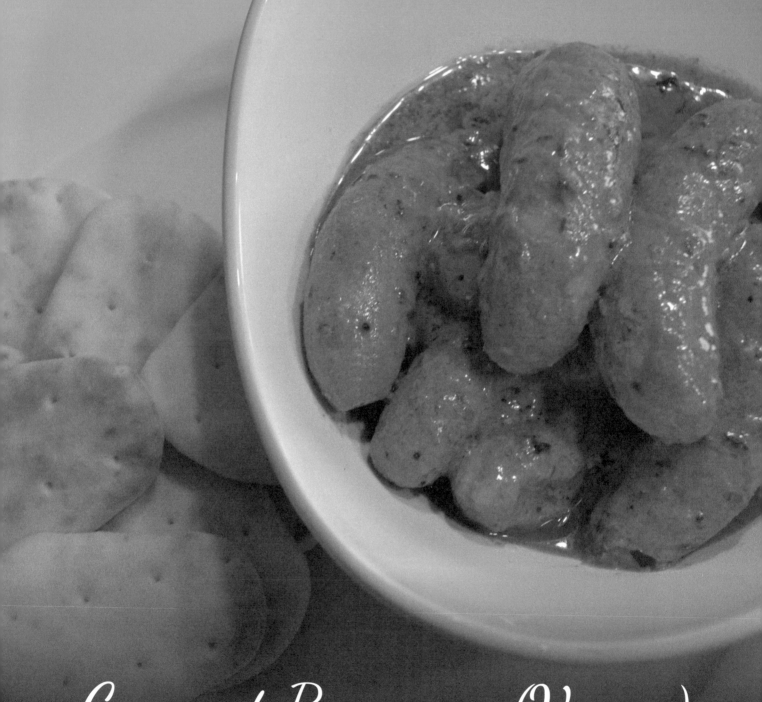

Coconut Bananas (Vegan)

Ingredients

8 baby green & peeled bananas
4 tbsp coconut oil
1 tsp crushed cumin seeds
1 finely chopped green chili
½ tsp paprika powder
Salt to taste
1 freshly squeezed lemon
2 cup water
5 tsp coconut powder

Procedure

1. Boil peeled bananas for 5 minutes on medium heat.
2. Heat oil in a pan; add bananas and rest of ingredients.
3. Cook on medium heat for 10 minutes and then for another 10 -15 minutes on low heat, stirring occasionally.

Serves 4-6

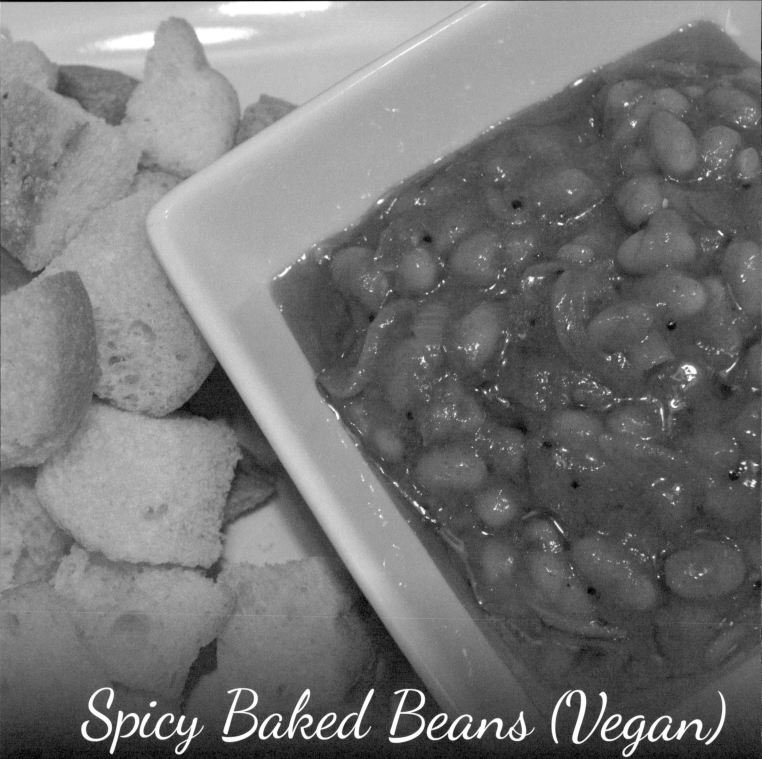

Spicy Baked Beans (Vegan)

Ingredients

2 cans of Heinz baked beans
1 cup chopped onions
¼ cup cooking oil
½ tsp mustard seeds
½ tsp turmeric powder
Salt to taste
½ cup water

Procedure

1. In a pan heat oil and add mustard seeds and onions.
2. Stir fry onions until light golden brown and add rest of ingredients.
3. Mix well and cook for 10-15 minutes

Serves 2-4

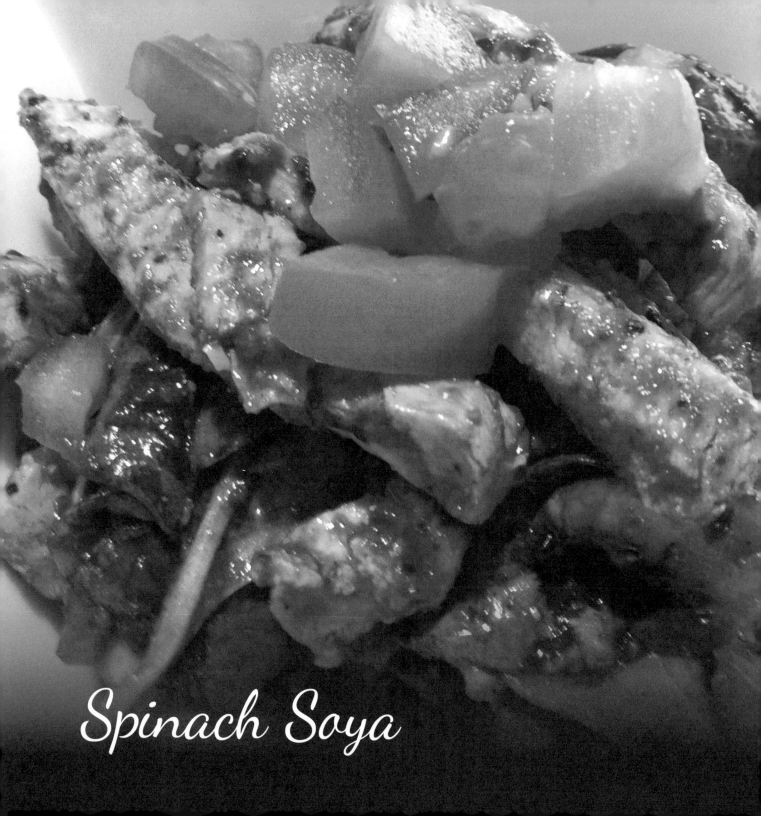

Spinach Soya

Ingredients

4 cups soya strips
¼ cup olive oil
2 cloves crushed garlic
½ lb. fresh spinach
¼ tsp. paprika powder
¼ cup water
2 tsp. fajita seasoning
1 large diced tomato

Procedure

1. Heat oil in pan and add soya strips and garlic. Stir well and cook for 3 minutes.
2. Add spinach, paprika, fajita seasoning, and water and cook 7–10 minutes more, stirring occasionally.
3. Remove from heat.
4. Add diced tomatoes before serving

Serves 4-6

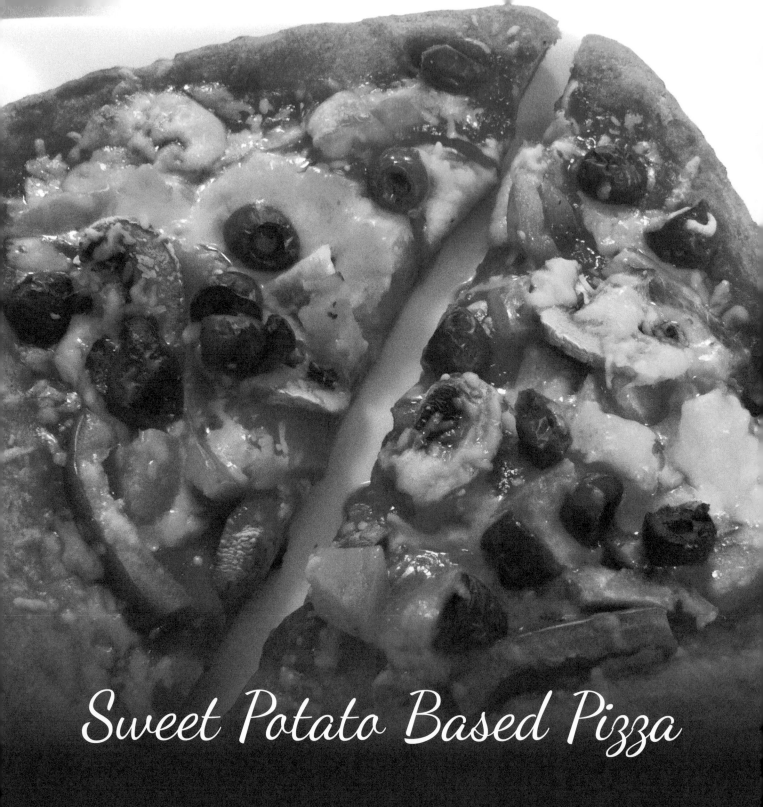

Sweet Potato Based Pizza

Ingredients for pizza base

2 cups wheat flour

2 cups boiled & mashed sweet potatoes

1 tsp fast action yeast

Three 8 inches x 8 inches aluminum foil trays

Ingredients for topping

1 cup tinned tomatoes

½ cup tomato paste

2 tsp mixed herbs

5 medium size sliced mushrooms,

2 diced fresh tomatoes

½ chopped green bell pepper

½ cup sliced olives,

1 cup grated cheese

Procedure

1. Mix and bind ingredients for pizza base in a bowl. Leave aside for 15 minutes for a good raise.
2. Grease the foil trays with oil.
3. Make three equal portions of the pizza base and spread them in the foil trays with finger tips.
4. Put tinned tomatoes, tomato paste and mixed herbs in a blender. Mix well to make the paste.
5. Spread the paste with a spoon on the pizza bases.
6. Sprinkle rest of the ingredients equally on the pizza bases.
7. Bake pizzas for 15-20 minutes at 400 °F (until golden brown).

Serves 2-3

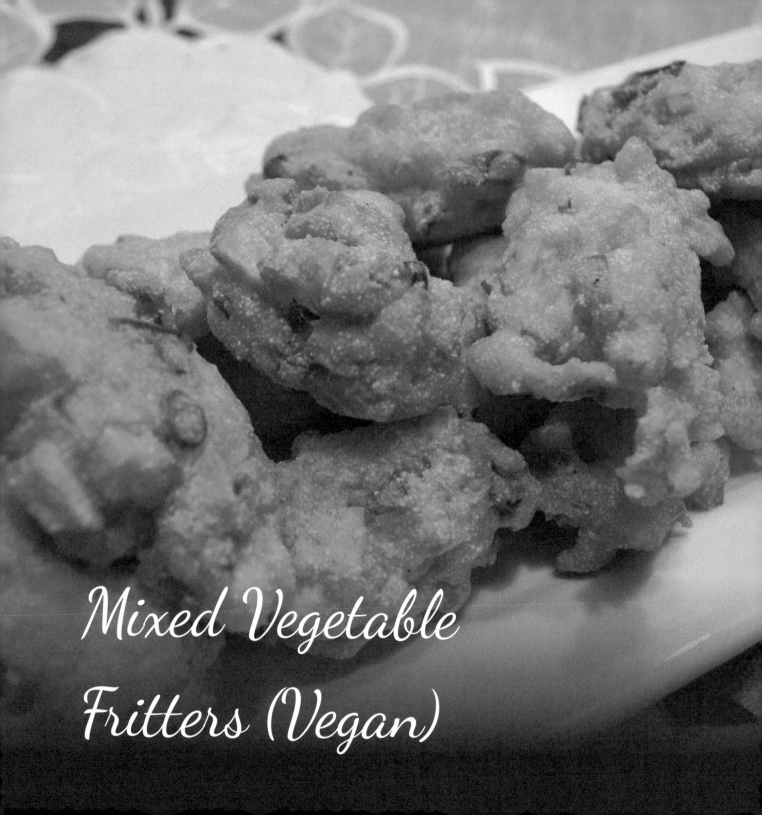

Mixed Vegetable Fritters (Vegan)

Ingredients

2cups chopped potatoes
½ cup diced green bell peppers
2cups corn flour
½ cup semolina
2 finely chopped green chilies
Salt to taste
2 tsp sugar
½ tsp baking powder
¼ tsp turmeric powder
½ freshly squeezed lemon
1 ¾ cups water
Oil for deep frying

Procedure

1. Mix well all the ingredients in a bowl.
2. Heat oil in a wok for deep frying.
3. With a table spoon drop the mixture one by one gently n the heated oil.
4. Fry, turning occasionally until golden brown.
5. Can be used as a starter.

Serves 5-6

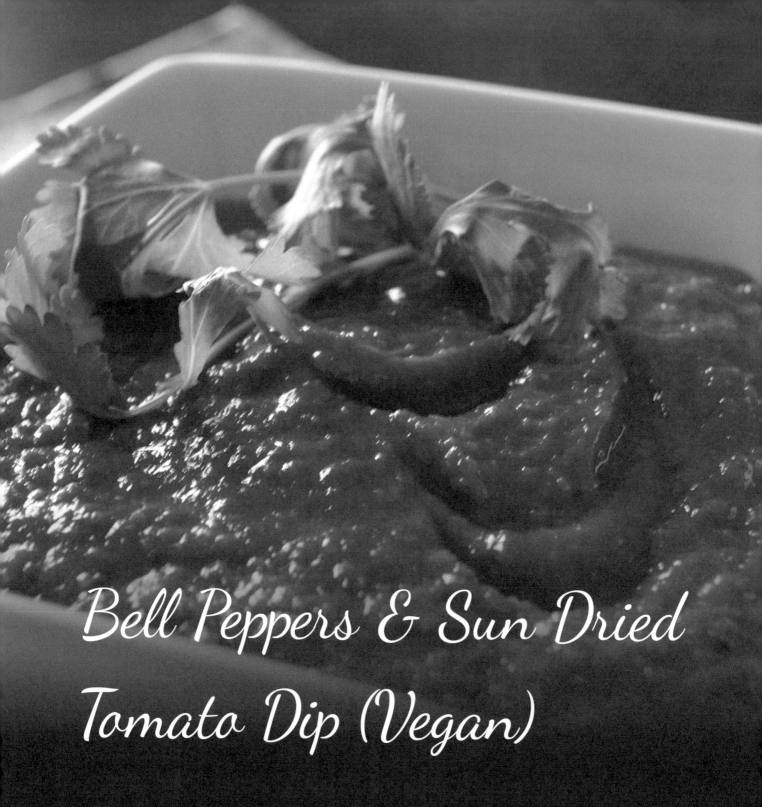

Bell Peppers & Sun Dried Tomato Dip (Vegan)

Ingredients

1 large red bell pepper
1 large tomato
½ cup sun dried tomatoes
3 cloves garlic
2 tsp sugar or sweetener
1 tsp salt (optional)
5 tbsp lemon juice
2 tsp red chili powder

Procedure

1. Put all ingredients in an electric mixer.
2. Crush until it is thoroughly pureed.

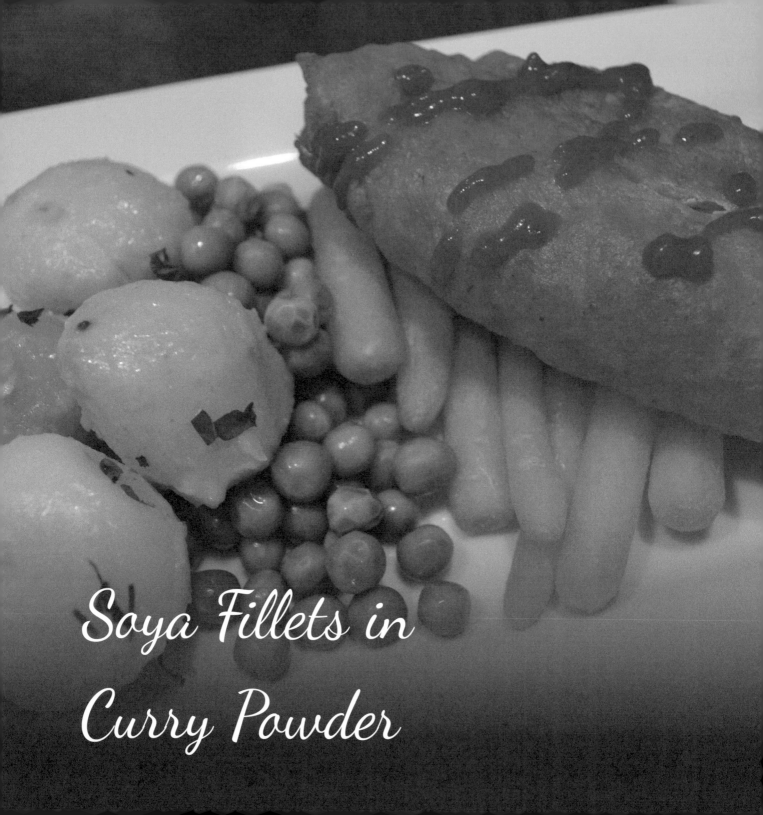

Soya Fillets in

Curry Powder

Ingredients

4 soya fillets
2 cups all-purpose flour
¼ cup corn starch
½ tsp baking powder
¼ tsp soda
2 tsp curry powder
¾ cup water
Oil for deep frying

Method

1. To make batter add flour, corn starch, baking powder, soda, curry powder, water in a bowl and mix well.
2. Dip fillets in batter and deep fry until crispy and golden brown.
3. Can be enjoyed with vegetables or rice.

Serves 4

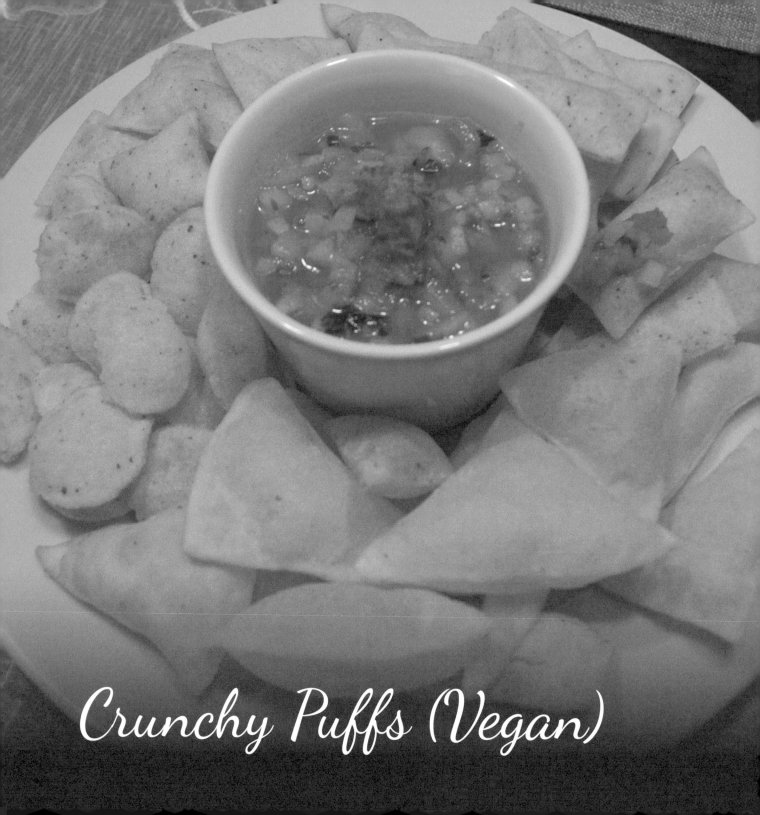

Crunchy Puffs (Vegan)

Ingredients

1cup semolina
2½ tsp crushed garlic
½ tsp oregano
½ cup water
Pinch of salt
Oil for deep frying

Procedure

1. In a bowl, combine semolina, garlic, oregano, water, salt and to make a dough.
2. Leave dough aside for half hour and divide into four equal portions.
3. Roll each portion on a flat surface and cut into shapes of your choice.
4. Deep fry the pieces in heated oil until puffed and golden brown.

Can be served as an appetizer or party snack. Goes well with any salsa.

Serves 6–8

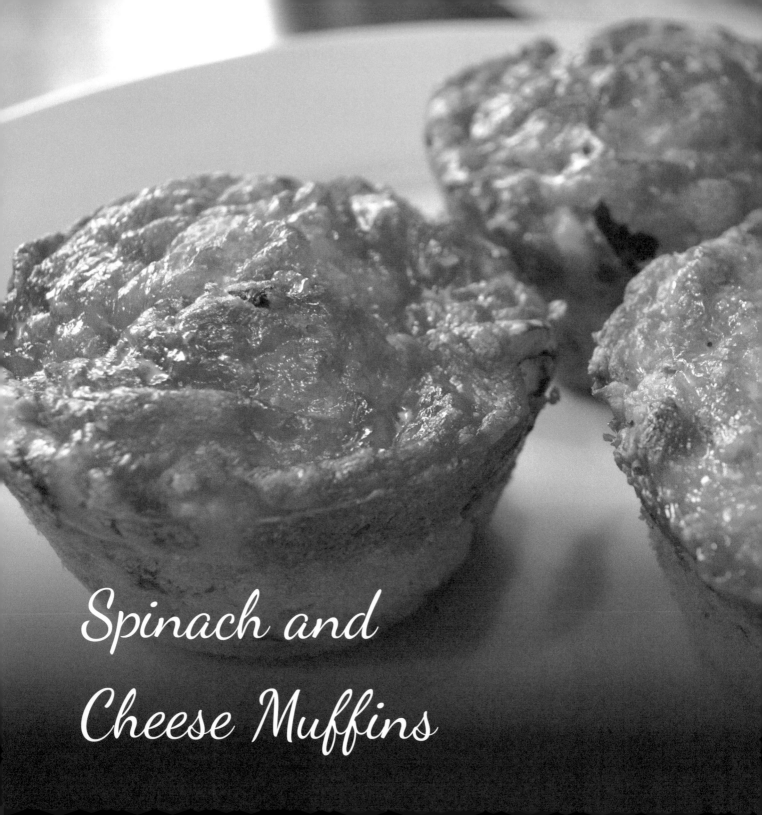

Spinach and
Cheese Muffins

Ingredients

2cups pancake flour
1 cup chopped spinach
½ cup grated cheddar cheese
½ cup crushed pepper
¾ cup water
½ cup grated cheddar cheese to sprinkle on top of muffins

Procedure

1. In a bowl, mix spinach, ½ cup cheese, crushed pepper and water.
2. Pour mixture in a muffin tray.
3. Sprinkle remaining ½ cup cheese on top of the mixture.
4. Bake in pre-heated oven at 400 °F for about 20 minutes.

Makes 4-6

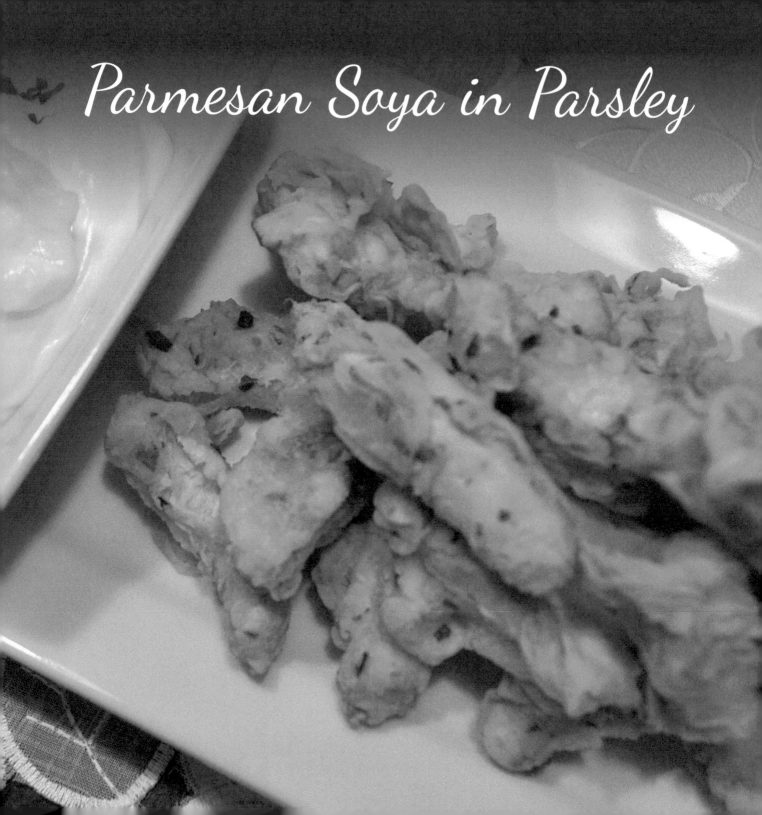

Parmesan Soya in Parsley

Ingredients

2cups soya strips
1 ½ cup all-purpose flour
1 tsp baking soda
2 tbsp parmesan cheese
1 ¾ cups water, salt to taste
1 tsp crushed black pepper
½ cup chopped parsley
1 tbsp lemon juice
1 cup all-purpose flour
oil for deep frying.

For dip: 1 cup sour cream, ½ tsp crushed garlic and
1 tsp parsley. Goes well with soya strips

Procedure

1. To make batter add all ingredients (except the soya strips and one cup flour) in a bowl and mix well.
2. Dip each strip in batter then into dry flour.
3. Deep fry until golden brown.
4. Can be served as finger food.

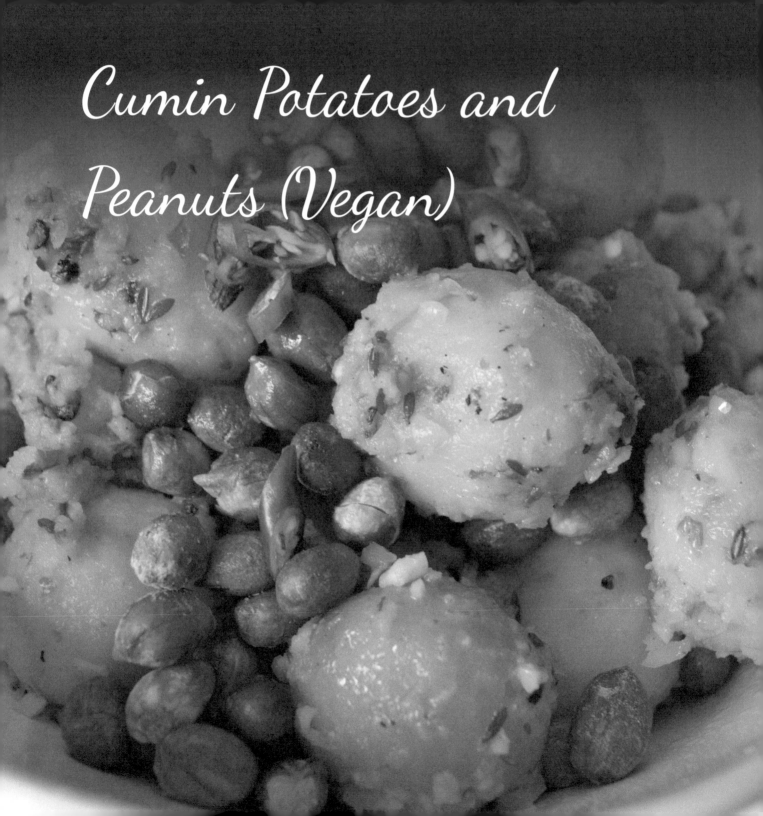

Cumin Potatoes and Peanuts (Vegan)

Ingredients

5 cups boiled and peeled baby potatoes
1/3 cup coconut oil, 1 tsp cumin seeds,
¼ cup shelled and crushed peanuts
¼ cup water, salt to taste
½ tsp crushed black pepper
2 tbsp lemon juice
½ cup peanuts for garnishing.

Procedure

1. Heat oil in a pan and add cumin seeds.
2. Add rest of ingredients and cook for 5-10 minutes.
3. Serve and garnish with peanuts.

Serves 4

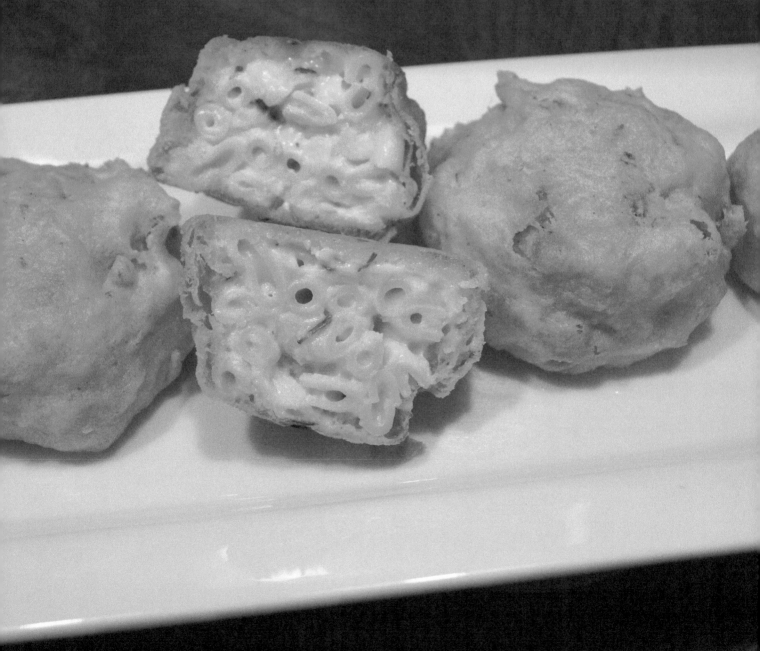

Mac & Cheese Bites

Ingredients

White sauce
(2 ½ cups milk
¼ cup butter
1 tbsp crushed garlic
1 tsp English mustard
½ cup white flour
1 cup water
½ cup grated cheddar cheese)
5 cups boiled elbow pasta

Procedure

1. In a pan, add milk, butter, mustard and bring to boil.
2. In a separate container add water, flour, mix well and slowly add to the pan making sure there are no lumps.
3. Added grated cheese and the boiled pasta. Allow to cool.
4. In a tray, make balls using a scoop and freeze them.

   Batter: 2 ¼ cups all-purpose flour, 2 ¼ cups water, ¼ cup corn starch, ¼ cup curry powder, 1 tsp fresh garlic, 2 tbsp crushed green chilies, 2 tsp baking powder, oil for deep frying.

5. Deep fry each of the frozen balls dipping them in batter and until golden brown

Makes 8-10

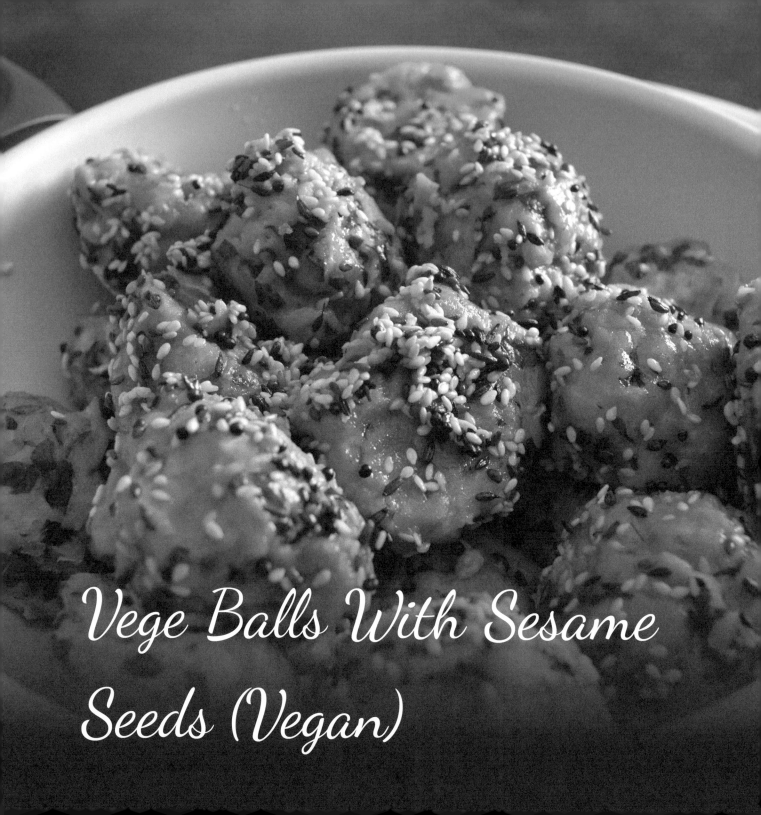

Vege Balls With Sesame Seeds (Vegan)

Ingredients

2cups wheat flour
2 cups grated zucchini
2 cups baby spinach
1 tsp turmeric powder
Salt to taste
1 tsp grated ginger
1tsp baking powder
¼ cup vegetable oil
½ to ¾ cup water.

For garnish: 4 tbsp vegetable oil, 3 tbsp of sesame seeds

Procedure

1. Put all the ingredients in a bowl and mix well.
2. Using hands make balls of approx. 1½ inches diameter.
3. Put the balls in a steamer for about 15 minutes to cook.
4. Transfer them into a bowl.
5. Heat oil in a pan and add sesame seeds to make the garnish.
6. Pour garnish onto the steamed vege balls.

Can be served as finger food.

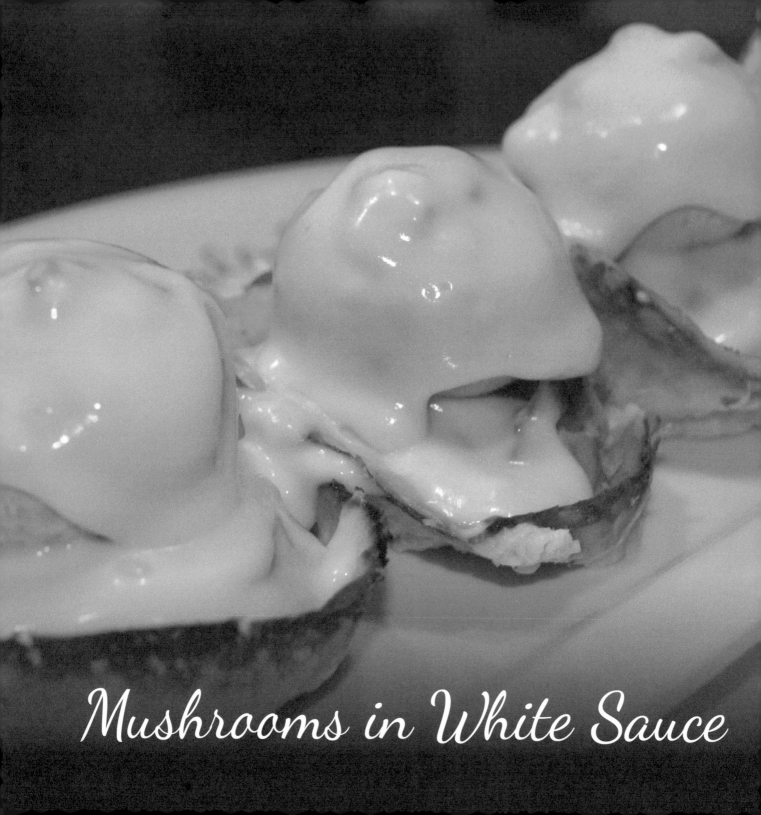
Mushrooms in White Sauce

Ingredients

12 white mushrooms
White sauce (2 ½ cups milk, ¼ cup butter,1 tsp English mustard,
½ cup white flour, 1 cup water, ½ cup cheddar cheese)
1 cup grated mozzarella cheese to sprinkle on mushrooms.

Procedure

1. In a pan, add milk, butter, mustard and bring to boil.
2. In a separate container add water, flour, mix well and slowly add to the pan making sure there are no lumps.
3. In a muffin tray pour white sauce and place mushrooms.
4. Add extra sauce on top of mushroom then top it with grated mozzarella cheese.
5. Bake in pre-heated oven at 400 °F for 15-20 minutes.

Serves 6

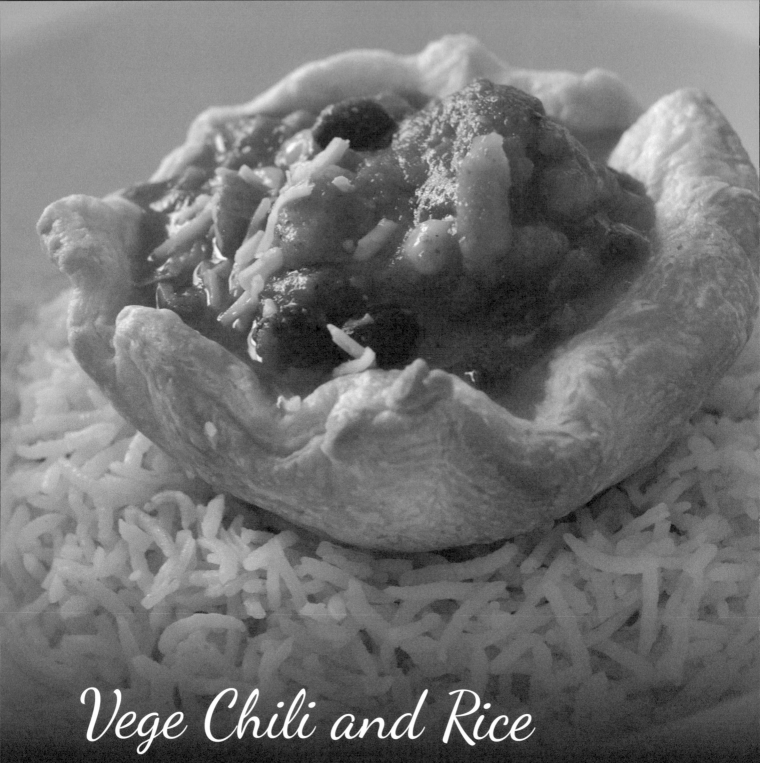

Vege Chili and Rice

Ingredients

1 cup minced soya
1 cup mixed vegetables
1 cup canned black beans
1cup canned kidney beans
1 cup canned tomatoes
¼ cup canned tomato paste
1 cup water
salt to taste

1 tsp coriander powder,
1 tsp cumin powder
1 tsp paprika powder
2tbsp cooking oil,
chilies to taste,
2 tbsp grated parmesan cheese
½ cup grated cheddar cheese for serving
1 roll pastry sheet.

Procedure

1. Cut 4 pieces of rolled pastry sheets (each approx. 6 inches diameter).
2. Turn a large muffin tray upside down.
3. Place each pastry sheet over the tray to give a boat shape and bake for about 15 minutes at 350 °F until it is golden brown and leave them on one side.
4. In a saucepan add minced soya, mixed vegetables, black beans, kidney beans, tomatoes, tomato paste, water, salt, coriander powder, cumin powder, paprika powder and cooking oil, chilies.
5. Cook on medium heat thoroughly while stirring occasionally.
6. Add parmesan cheese and mix well.
7. Serve chili in the pastry placed on a bed of boiled rice.

Serves 4

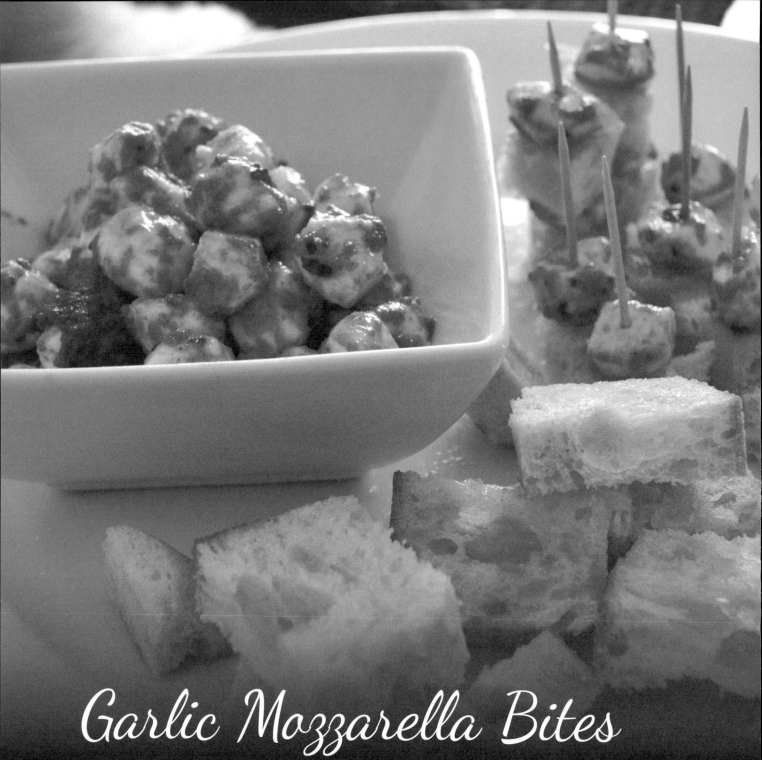

Garlic Mozzarella Bites

Ingredients

1 ½ cup diced mozzarela cheese
1 clove crushed garlic
1 tsp flaked red pepper
1 tsp papprika powder
½ cup olive

Procedure

1. Add crushed garlic, red pepper, paprprika powder, and olive oil in a mixer and make a chutney.
2. In a small container pour chutney over the diced cheese and mix well.

Best eaten as a finger food with any bread

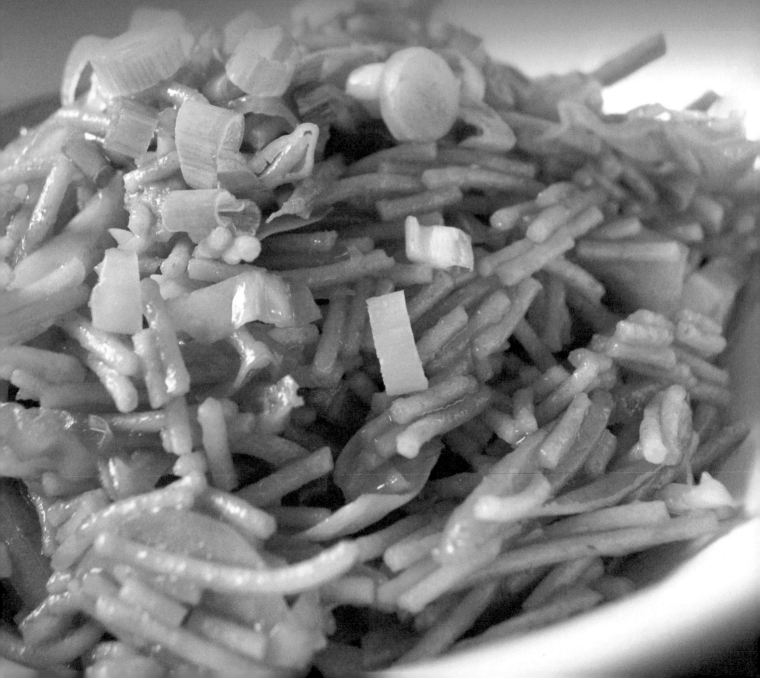
Vege Noodles (Vegan)

Ingredients

4 cups boiled thin noodles
1 cup shreded carrots
1 cup chopped peppers
½ cup chopped spring onions
¼ cup oil
2 tsp crushed garlic
¾ cup ketchup
A dash of paprika powder
¼ cup soya sauce
1tsp sesame seed oil

Method

1. Heat oil in a pan and add garlic, ¼ cup spring onions, ketchup, paprika powder, soya sauce.
2. Stir and cook for 3 minutes .
3. Add noodles, carrots, peppers and rest of spring onions and mix well.
4. Cook for 3 minutes on medium heat, add sesame seed oil and mix gently.

Serves 2-4

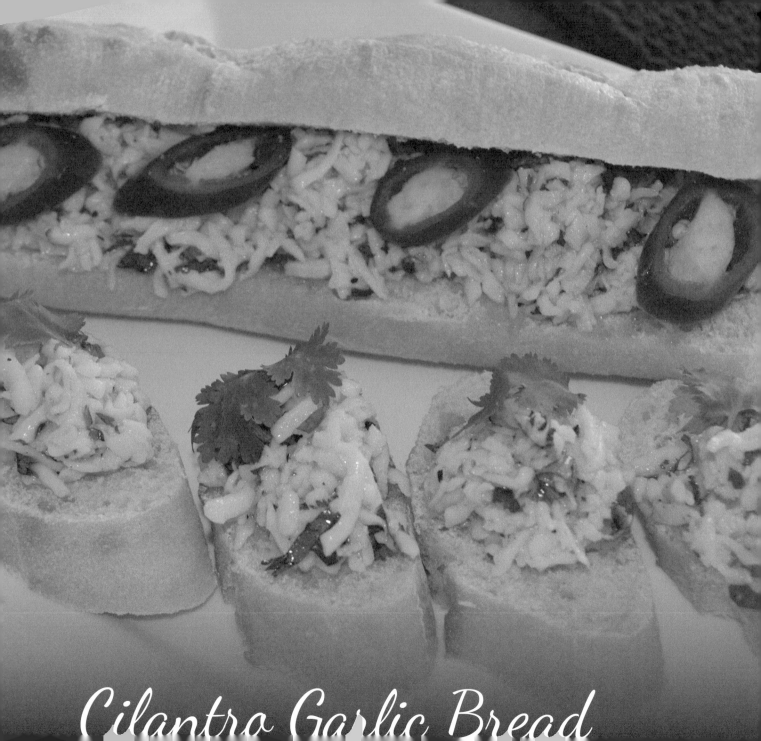

Cilantro Garlic Bread

Ingredients

2 cups cilantro
½ cup olive oil
1 jalapeno
Salt to taste
1 cup diced mozzarella cheese
1 stick of bread

Procedure

1. Add cilantro, olive oil, jalapeno and salt in a mixer and make a chutney.
2. In a small container pour chutney over the diced cheese and mix well.
3. Cut bread stick from centre and transfer cubes of cheese.
4. Place the bread stick in the oven for 10 to 15 minutes in a pre heated oven on gas mark 400 °F.

Serves 4

Potato Fritters (Vegan)

Ingredients

2 large potatoes
½ cup corn flour
½ cup gram flour
¼ tsp turmeric powder
2 tsp sugar or sweetener
2 tbsp lemon juice
½ cup cilantro
Salt to taste
¼ to ½ cup water
Oil for deep frying

Procedure

1. Peel potatoes and make about 2 mm thick slices
2. In a bowl, add all ingredients and mix well
3. Fry slices of the battered potatoes until golden brown.
4. Serve with a dip of your choice (finger food).

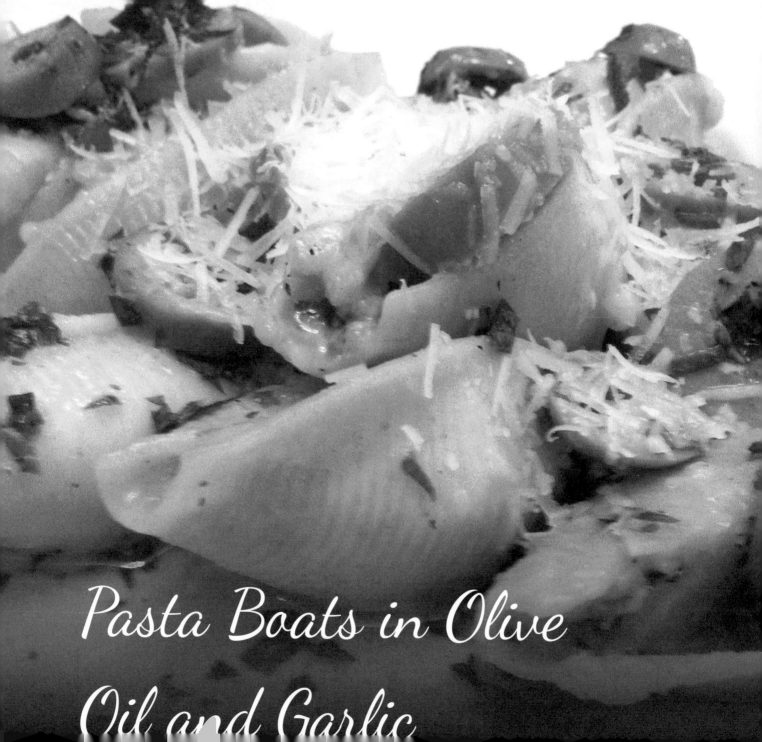

Pasta Boats in Olive Oil and Garlic

Ingredients

3cups barley
1 cup ricotta cheese
1 cup freshly chopped parsley,
1 tsp flaked pepper,
½ tsp black pepper

¼ cup water
salt to taste,
2 tsp soft margarine
35 pasta shells.

Ingredients for garnishing olive oil

½ cup chopped parsley, 6 cloves crushed garlic, 2
cups olive oil, 2 cups sliced green olives

Procedure

a. For garnishing olive oil, mix all ingredients in a bowl and leave aside for serving.
b. Boil barley in a pan with 4 cups water for 15-20 minutes, Drain water.
c. In a mixing bowl put boiled barley, ricotta cheese, chopped parsley, flaked pepper, black pepper, salt, water, margarine and mix well. Leave aside.
d. In a pan put pasta shells in water and boil until cooked.
e. Drain water from pasta and let the pasta to cool down.
f. Stuff pasta shells with the barley mixture and leave aside.
g. Heat stuffed pasta shells in a microwave for 5-7 minutes and remove.
h. Serve pasta shells with garnishing olive oil.

Serves 4

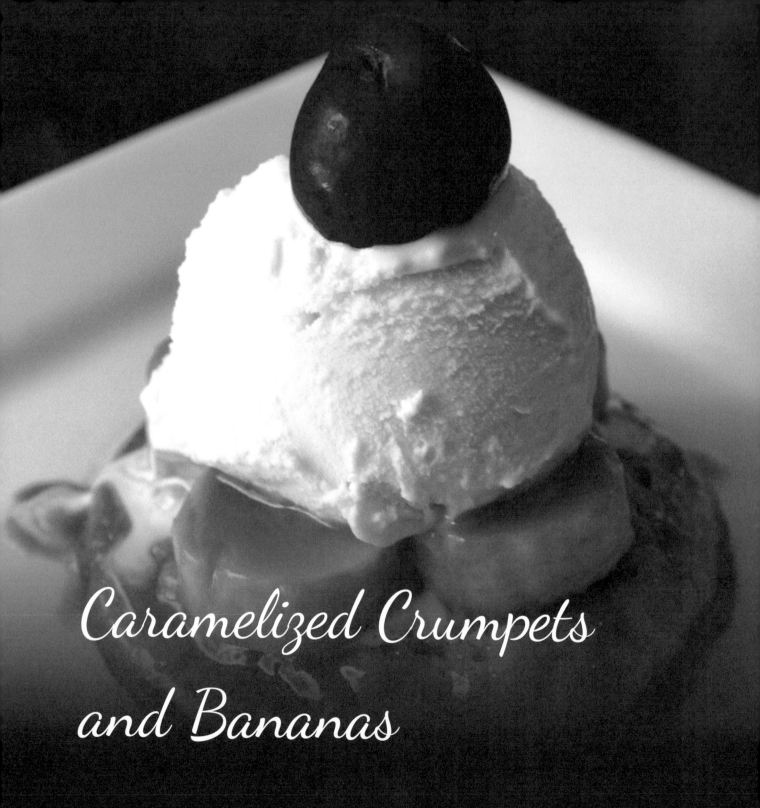

Caramelized Crumpets
and Bananas

Ingredients for caramel

½ cup sugar, 1 cup fresh cream, 2 tbsp butter

Method (for caramel)

1. In a pan add sugar and stir on medium heat.
2. Melt sugar until it turns golden brown.
3. Add cream, finally add butter and mix well.

Ingredients

4 crumpets, 4 chopped bananas, vanilla ice cream, 4 cherries

1. Toast crumpets and spread butter.
2. Place crumpet on a serving plate.
3. Add chopped bananas and drizzle caramel with a spoon.
4. Top it up with a dollop of ice cream and cherry.

Serves 4

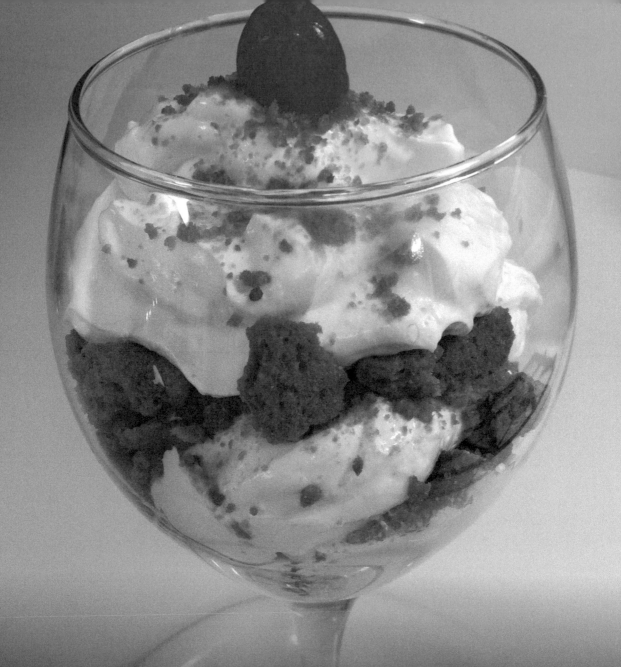

Fluffy Cheesecake

Ingredients

1 cup soft white cheese
1 ½ cups heavy whipping cream
½ cup powdered sugar
8-10 crumbled ginger snaps
4 glazed cherries

Procedure

1. In a bowl, add soft cheese, cream and sugar.
2. Mix well to make into a cheese cake mix.
3. Prepare 4 glasses to serve.
4. In each glass make layers of cheese cake and crumbled ginger snaps.
5. Top each serving with a cherry.

Serves 4

Printed in the United States
By Bookmasters